M. A. DAVIS

Healthy Living for the Midlife Woman

Exercising and Eating Healthy on a Budget

This book was professionally typeset on Reedsy.
Find out more at reedsy.com

Contents

1

Introduction

Welcome to "Healthy Living for the Midlife Woman: Exercising and Eating Healthy on a Budget." I'm here to guide you through the twists and turns of midlife, not as an expert, but as someone who's there and found a path worth sharing. Why? Because I know simple changes can transform your life without draining your bank account.

As we get older it gets harder and harder to lose weight, and then keep it off. We struggle with finding and keeping our motivation, and we barely have enough energy to make it through the day, let alone think about trying to exercise and eat right. Even if we did have the motivation and energy, where would we find the extra hours needed to start exercising and eating healthy?

This book will be ideal for women in their 40s and 50s who want to lose some weight, get in better shape, and live a healthier lifestyle. This is not a diet book, diets are short-term fixes, that typically do not bring about lifelong changes, this book is meant to be a guide for a new way of life.

I am hoping that this book will be the starting point for you and provide you with the platform that you need to start making better life choices and find the healthier happier midlife you! You will learn how to implement a simple workout routine in the comfort of your own home without having to purchase expensive exercise equipment that will just end up taking up space in your home. You will also learn how to eat healthy on a budget and how to develop a routine to help you continue with your new healthier lifestyle.

In the pages ahead, we're diving into practical home exercise plans that won't cost a fortune. No need for pricey gym memberships or fancy gear. We're also tackling eating well on a budget, proving that healthy doesn't have to mean expensive. This book isn't about miracles; it's about real, doable shifts that fit your budget, your schedule, and your desire for a healthier you.

So, let's get down to it. Flip to Chapter 2, "Getting Active," where we kick off the real action. No fluff, just a roadmap to a healthier, happier you. Join me, as we navigate midlife together, making vitality a practical and budget-friendly part of your life.

2

Getting Active

W elcome to the health frontier! In this chapter, we'll unravel the perks of staying active as you navigate midlife. No gym fees or complicated equipment needed—just practical tips and routines to keep you moving.

Benefits of Staying Active in Midlife

Let's cut to the chase—why bother staying active? Staying active in midlife isn't just about breaking a sweat; it's a game-changer for your health. Regular activity is like a superhero cape, defending against a host of issues. First up, it's a mood booster, releasing those feel-good chemicals that combat stress and elevate your spirits. But that's not all. Keep moving, and you're giving your heart a solid ally, reducing the risk of heart disease. Your bones join the party too, staying strong and resilient. Active living isn't just a workout; it's a shield against weight gain, helping you maintain a healthy body. And let's not forget the energy boost—it's like your personal power-up, keeping you vibrant and ready for whatever life throws your way. Being active isn't a chore; it's an investment in your health and it's not about complicated routines;

it's about making movement a regular part of your life. So, get moving, and let your health reap the rewards of a more active lifestyle.

Simple Tricks to Add More Movement into Everyday Life

Exercise doesn't always mean hitting the gym. Discover easy hacks to sneak more movement into your daily routine. It's the small, practical changes that add up. First off, park your car in the furthest spot when you hit the store. Those extra steps make a difference. Elevators and escalators? Swap them for the stairs. It's an instant boost for your legs and a simple way to sneak in more movement.

Next up, let's talk about screen time. Break it up with quick bursts of activity. For every hour you sit, take a five-minute stroll or stretch. It's like hitting a reset button for your body. And hey, don't underestimate the power of a good old-fashioned walk. If it's a short distance, ditch the car and walk—it's not just eco-friendly; it's body-friendly too.

Now, let's tackle the sitting trap. Set a timer to remind yourself to stand up and move around every 30 minutes. A quick stretch or a stroll around the office can do wonders. And don't forget the magic of multitasking— do some squats while you brush your teeth or calf raises while waiting for your coffee to brew.

The goal here isn't a radical overhaul; it's about integrating movement naturally. These uncomplicated tweaks may seem small, but their cumulative effect is significant. So, let's keep it practical and achievable—add more steps, take those stairs, and make movement an organic part of your everyday life. Your body will appreciate the subtle shift.

30-Minute or Less Home Workout Routines

Busy schedule? No problem. Dive into workout routines that won't devour your day—30 minutes or less is all you need. Say goodbye to excuses and hello to effective, time-efficient workouts. No equipment is needed, just dedication and a little bit of space.

Week 1: Full Body Basics

Day 1:

- Warm-up (5 minutes): Brisk walk or jog in place
- Main Workout (20 minutes):
- Bodyweight squats
- Push-ups (modify using a wall or countertop)
- Cool Down (5 minutes): Stretching

Day 2:

- Warm-up (5 minutes): Jumping jacks
- Main Workout (20 minutes):
- Lunges (alternate legs)
- Plank holds
- Cool Down (5 minutes): Relaxation stretches

Day 3:

- Warm-up (5 minutes): Dynamic stretches
- Main Workout (20 minutes):
- Jumping squats
- Tricep push-ups
- Cool Down (5 minutes): Deep breathing exercises

Day 4:

- Warm-up (5 minutes): High knees
- Main Workout (20 minutes):
- Side lunges
- Bicycle crunches
- Cool Down (5 minutes): Gentle stretches

Keep the momentum going, adjusting intensity and pace as needed.

Week 2: Cardio Blast

Day 1:

- Warm-up (5 minutes): High knees
- Main Workout (25 minutes):
- Dancing or aerobics
- Burpees
- Cool Down (5 minutes): Gentle stretches

Day 2:

- Warm-up (5 minutes): Mountain climbers
- Main Workout (25 minutes):
- Jumping rope
- Bicycle crunches
- Cool Down (5 minutes): Deep breathing exercises

Day 3:

- Warm-up (5 minutes): Running in place
- Main Workout (25 minutes):
- Jumping jacks
- Plank to downward dog

- Cool Down (5 minutes): Relaxation poses

Day 4:

- Warm-up (5 minutes): High knees
- Main Workout (25 minutes):
- Box jumps (or step-ups)
- Mountain climbers
- Cool Down (5 minutes): Stretching

Add some zest to your routine and adjust based on your energy levels.

Week 3: Core Focus

Day 1:

- Warm-up (5 minutes): Jog in place
- Main Workout (25 minutes):
- Russian twists
- Leg raises
- Cool Down (5 minutes): Gentle stretches

Day 2:

- Warm-up (5 minutes): Side plank (each side)
- Main Workout (25 minutes):
- Bicycle crunches
- Flutter kicks
- Cool Down (5 minutes): Relaxation poses

Day 3:

- Warm-up (5 minutes): High knees
- Main Workout (25 minutes):
- Plank rotations
- Superman holds
- Cool Down (5 minutes): Deep breathing exercises

Day 4:

- Warm-up (5 minutes): Dynamic stretches
- Main Workout (25 minutes):
- Mountain climbers
- Russian twists
- Cool Down (5 minutes): Stretching

Focus on building core strength, alternating routines throughout the week.

Week 4: Mix It Up

Day 1:

- Warm-up (5 minutes): Jump squats
- Main Workout (30 minutes):
- Dance workout
- Tricep dips (use a sturdy chair)
- Cool Down (5 minutes): Stretching

Day 2:

- Warm-up (5 minutes): Burpees
- Main Workout (30 minutes):
- High knees

- Plank to push-up transitions
- Cool Down (5 minutes): Deep breathing exercises

Day 3:

- Warm-up (5 minutes): Jumping jacks
- Main Workout (30 minutes):
- Bodyweight squats
- Bicycle crunches
- Cool Down (5 minutes): Gentle stretches

Day 4:

- Warm-up (5 minutes): High knees
- Main Workout (30 minutes):
- Lunges (alternate legs)
- Plank holds
- Cool Down (5 minutes): Relaxation stretches

Rotate exercises to keep it interesting and maintain the challenge. Consistency is key—keep moving! Feel free to personalize and swap exercises based on your preferences and fitness level. Consistency is the game-changer here, so stay committed and enjoy the benefits of these quick and effective home workouts. You've got this!

Workout Routines if You Have Back or Knee Issues

When dealing with back or knee issues, exercise becomes a delicate balancing act between staying active and preventing further strain. Let's dive into practical workout routines that prioritize strengthening these areas while minimizing impact. If you have any concerns about starting a workout routine consult with your doctor.

<u>Back-Friendly Exercises</u>

    1. Cat-Cow Stretch:

- Begin on hands and knees.
- Arch your back like a cat, then dip it down like a cow.
- Repeat for 10 cycles, promoting flexibility and strength in the spine.

2. Partial Crunches:

- Lie on your back with knees bent.
- Lift your head and shoulders off the ground, engaging your core.
- Focus on controlled movements to avoid straining your neck.

3. Swimming Exercise:

- Lie face down, extend arms, and lift opposite arm and leg.
- Keep movements deliberate to engage lower back muscles without excessive strain.

<u>Knee-Friendly Exercises</u>

    1. Wall Sits:

- Lean against a wall with knees at a 90-degree angle.
- Hold for 20-30 seconds, targeting quadriceps without stressing the knees.

2. Leg Raises:

- Lie on your back, lift one leg at a time without bending the knee.
- Engage your core to provide support to the lower back.

3. *Seated Knee Extensions:*

- Sit on a chair and straighten one leg at a time.
- Utilize a resistance band for added challenge without compromising knee integrity.

General Tips for Back and Knee Health

1. *Warm-Up:*

- Prioritize a gentle warm-up with dynamic stretches to prepare muscles for exercise, enhancing flexibility and reducing the risk of strain.

2. *Low-Impact Cardio:*

- Opt for low-impact cardio exercises such as swimming or cycling to provide cardiovascular benefits without exerting excessive pressure on the back and knees.

3. *Core Strengthening:*

- Cultivate a robust core, essential for supporting the back. Integrate exercises like planks and bridges to fortify core muscles.

4. *Listen to Your Body:*

- Pay close attention to how your body responds during exercise. If any movement induces pain, modify or omit that specific exercise. Pain is a signal to proceed with caution.

5. Gradual Progression:

- Initiate your routine with low-intensity exercises, gradually increasing intensity as your strength improves. Patience is key to avoiding setbacks.

Before embarking on any exercise program, particularly with existing back or knee concerns, seek guidance from a healthcare professional. This guide provides general advice, but individual conditions may vary. The journey to strengthening your back and knees is about steady progress and ensuring your well-being every step of the way.

3

Eating Healthy on a Budget

Get ready to transform your kitchen into a hub of nutritious and budget-friendly delights. This chapter is all about making healthy eating accessible, from smart shopping to effortless meal preparation and cooking delicious, wallet-friendly meals in 30 minutes.

Tips for Shopping for Low-Budget Healthy Eating:

Navigate the aisles with confidence as we unravel the secrets of budget-savvy shopping for nutritious meals. Discover how to maximize your grocery haul without breaking the bank, from choosing affordable yet nutrient-packed ingredients to making the most of sales and discounts. These practical tips empower you to make the most of your grocery budget, ensuring that you can fill your cart with nutritious options without overspending.

- Plan Before You Go: Map out your weekly meals and create a shopping list based on your needs. Sticking to your list prevents impulse buys and helps you stay focused on essentials.

- Buy in Bulk: Explore the bulk section for staples like rice, beans, and oats. Buying in larger quantities often comes with lower per-unit costs, making it a budget-friendly choice.

- Embrace Frozen and Canned Produce: Don't shy away from the frozen and canned aisles. These options, such as frozen vegetables or canned fruits, are not only economical but also have a longer shelf life, minimizing waste.

- Explore Store Brands: Generic or store brands offer quality comparable to name brands but at a lower price point. Take the time to compare labels and make informed choices.

- Hunt for Sales and Discounts: Keep an eye on weekly sales and discounts. Consider stocking up on non-perishable items when they are on special, maximizing your savings.

- Shop Seasonally: Align your meal plan with seasonal produce. Seasonal fruits and vegetables are often more affordable, and their freshness adds a delightful touch to your meals.

- Choose Cheaper Protein Sources: Opt for budget-friendly protein options such as eggs, canned tuna, chicken thighs, or legumes. These choices provide versatility and nutritional value without straining your budget.

- Minimize Processed Foods: Processed foods often come with a higher price tag. Stick to whole, unprocessed ingredients and embrace cooking from scratch whenever possible. It's not only cost-effective but also healthier.

- Be Mindful of Unit Prices: Scan the unit prices on shelf tags to make informed decisions. Sometimes, buying in larger quantities can be more economical, but it's essential to compare and evaluate.

- Don't Shop Hungry: Avoid the pitfalls of shopping on an empty stomach. Eating before heading to the store ensures you make mindful choices and resist the allure of impulse purchases.

Armed with these practical tips, your shopping experience transforms into a strategic mission, allowing you to stretch your budget while filling your cart with wholesome, nutritious choices.

Meal and Food Prep for a Beginner

Embark on your journey to healthy eating with foolproof meal and food prep strategies. We'll guide you through the basics of planning and prepping meals for the week, ensuring that nutritious choices are at your fingertips, even on your busiest days. Learn how to batch-cook staples and assemble meals with ease.

It doesn't require extensive experience or a kitchen full of gadgets. Here's a practical guide to simplify your cooking routine, minimize time investment, and maximize efficiency—all while using basic kitchen tools:

- Batch Cooking Basics: Dedicate a specific day for batch cooking to streamline your week. Prepare large quantities of staple ingredients like rice, quinoa, grilled chicken, or roasted veggies that can serve as the foundation for various meals.
- Optimize Ingredients: Choose ingredients that can multitask. Roast a variety of vegetables that can be incorporated into salads, wraps, or served as a side dish throughout the week.
- Extend Freshness with Proper Storage: Invest in basic storage containers with airtight seals to keep prepared ingredients fresh. Proper storage prevents food from drying out and maintains optimal taste.
- Utilize Leftovers Creatively: Embrace the art of transforming leftovers into new and exciting meals. For example, repurpose grilled

chicken into a salad or use roasted vegetables as a flavorful topping for a grain bowl.

- Plan for Versatile Ingredients: Opt for ingredients with versatility. Cook a large batch of quinoa or rice that can be used as a base for salads, grain bowls, or served as a side dish.
- Make Use of Freezer-Friendly Options: Leverage your freezer for long-term storage. Freeze portions of soups, stews, or cooked proteins for quick and easy future meals. Properly label and date items for easy identification.
- Cook Once, Eat Twice: Plan meals that share common ingredients to minimize prep time. If you're roasting sweet potatoes, use them in different dishes throughout the week to add variety without additional effort.
- Minimize Waste with Smart Shopping: Purchase fresh produce in quantities that align with your planned meals to avoid unnecessary spoilage. Choose pantry staple items that have a longer shelf life and can be used over time.
- Practice Safe Storage and Handling: Adhere to food safety guidelines to ensure the well-being of you and your family. Store raw meats separately, refrigerate leftovers promptly, and pay attention to expiration dates.

By following these beginner-friendly meal and food prep strategies, you'll find that navigating the kitchen becomes a more enjoyable and efficient experience. Embrace the joy of preparing meals ahead, making wholesome and delicious options readily available for your everyday enjoyment.

4

Cooking for Two - Easy, Affordable, and Healthy Meals in 30 Minutes

W elcome to the kitchen where simplicity meets health and affordability. This chapter is your go-to guide for mastering the art of preparing quick, delicious, and budget-friendly meals designed for at least two people. From cooking basics and helpful tips to reducing fat, calories, and sodium, to an array of easy and tasty recipes spanning breakfast, lunch, dinner, desserts, and snacks, we've got your culinary journey covered. This will make healthy eating a seamless part of your daily routine.

Cooking Basics: Tips and Tricks

Welcome to the foundation of your culinary journey. This section is designed to empower you with essential cooking knowledge, and time-saving tricks that will elevate your confidence in the kitchen.

- Knife Skills 101: Sharpen your knife skills for efficiency and safety. Learn proper techniques for chopping, dicing, and slicing to enhance the preparation of ingredients.

- Understanding Heat Levels: Grasp the nuances of heat levels on your stove. Whether simmering, boiling, or sauteing, knowing the right temperature for each cooking method is key to achieving perfect results.
- Balancing Flavors: Explore the art of flavor balancing. Understand how sweet, salty, sour, and bitter elements interact to create harmonious dishes. Experiment with seasoning to tailor flavors to your liking.
- Perfecting Pantry Essentials: Build a well-stocked pantry with essential ingredients. Having basics like herbs, spices, oils, and grains at your fingertips enhances your ability to create flavorful and varied dishes.
- Versatile Cooking Techniques: Master versatile cooking techniques like sauteing, roasting, and braising. Understanding these methods opens up a world of possibilities for preparing diverse and delicious meals.
- Safe Food Handling: Prioritize food safety with proper handling techniques. From storing ingredients to preventing cross-contamination, ensure that your kitchen practices promote a healthy and safe cooking environment.
- Detailed Prep: Take the time to chop, measure, and organize ingredients before cooking. Having everything ready ensures a smooth and efficient process in the kitchen.
- Efficiency Hack: Invest in small bowls or containers to organize prepped ingredients. This minimizes clutter and makes it easy to grab and add items to the cooking process swiftly.
- Sharp Tools: Keep your knives sharp; a sharp knife makes cutting easier and safer. Consider investing in a knife sharpener to maintain blade precision.
- Invest in Quality Tools: Invest in quality kitchen tools. Prioritize a sharp chef's knife for versatility, a durable cutting board to protect

your knives, and reliable cookware that distributes heat evenly.

- Care and Maintenance: Learn proper care and maintenance for your tools. Regularly sharpen knives, season cast iron pans, and follow care instructions to extend the life of your kitchen equipment.

- Create a Flavor Base: Master the technique of sauteing onions, garlic, and spices. This simple step at the beginning of your recipes builds a flavor foundation for your dishes.

- Experimentation: Experiment with different combinations of aromatics to discover unique flavor profiles. Don't shy away from trying new spices and herbs to elevate your dishes.

- Embrace Sheet Pan Cooking: Experiment with a variety of sheet pan recipes. It's a versatile method for cooking proteins, veggies, and even grains simultaneously.

- Parchment Paper Hack: Use parchment paper for easy cleanup. This not only prevents sticking but also makes washing up a breeze.

- Master One-Pot Wonders: Embrace the convenience of one-pot meals where flavors meld together. Stews, casseroles, and pasta dishes become delicious and time-saving.

- Adapt Recipes: Experiment with adapting your favorite recipes into one-pot wonders. Simplify the process without compromising on taste.

- Learn the Art of Batch Cooking: Plan your meals for the week and batch cook staple ingredients. This strategic approach saves time on daily cooking and ensures you always have a quick meal option.

- Freezing Tips: Understand proper freezing techniques to maintain the quality of batch-cooked meals. Invest in quality freezer-safe containers to avoid freezer burn.

- Clever Ingredient Substitutions: Be open to ingredient substitutions based on availability. Greek yogurt can replace sour cream, and olive oil can stand in for butter in certain recipes.

- Taste Testing: Always taste-test when substituting ingredients to ensure the flavor profile aligns with your preferences.

- Clean As You Go: Develop a habit of cleaning as you go. Wipe down surfaces and wash utensils during downtimes to maintain a tidy workspace.
- Post-Meal Soaking: Soak pans immediately after use to simplify post-meal cleanup. This eases the removal of stuck-on food.
- Kitchen Cheat Sheet: Create a cheat sheet with common conversions and keep it in your kitchen for quick reference. This ensures accuracy when following recipes.
- Lastly, embrace your creativity in the kitchen. Don't be afraid to experiment with flavors, try new recipes, and adapt dishes to suit your preferences. Cooking is an art, and the kitchen is your canvas.

Incorporating these detailed tips and tricks into your cooking routine empowers you with practical skills, making your time in the kitchen more efficient, enjoyable, and successful.

Ways to Reduce Fat, Calories, Sugar, and Sodium When You Cook

Explore practical strategies to make your meals healthier without sacrificing flavor. Below are some useful techniques to cut down on fat, calories, and sodium while maintaining the deliciousness of your dishes.

Good Fat vs. Bad Fat:

- Good Fats: Opt for sources of monounsaturated and polyunsaturated fats like avocados, nuts, seeds, and olive oil. These fats contribute to heart health, provide essential fatty acids, and help absorb fat-soluble vitamins.
- Limit Saturated Fats: Reduce saturated fats found in butter, fatty

cuts of meat, and full-fat dairy. Choose leaner protein options, like poultry or fish, and use olive oil or canola oil for cooking.

Lower Calorie Substitutes:

- Veggies as Base: Incorporate more vegetables into your meals, either as a main component or by substituting some meat with veggies. Mushrooms, lentils, or beans are excellent choices to reduce calorie density while adding fiber and nutrients.
- Greek Yogurt: Replace sour cream or mayonnaise with Greek yogurt in recipes. It maintains creaminess with fewer calories and adds a protein boost to your dishes.

Reduced Sugar Options:

- Natural Sweeteners: Opt for natural sweeteners like honey, maple syrup, or agave nectar. While moderation is key, these alternatives provide sweetness with additional nutrients compared to refined sugar.
- Fruit Puree: Use fruit purees, such as applesauce or mashed bananas, in baking to reduce the need for added sugar. They contribute natural sweetness and moisture to recipes.

Low Sodium Alternatives:

- Herbs and Spices: Enhance flavor with herbs and spices instead of salt. Experiment with garlic, cumin, paprika, or rosemary to add depth without the sodium. Herbs also provide additional health benefits.
- Homemade Broth: Make your own broth using vegetables, herbs, and lean meat to control sodium content. This ensures a flavorful

base for your recipes without relying on high-sodium store-bought options.

Lean Protein Choices:

- Poultry and Fish: Choose lean protein sources like chicken or turkey breast and fish. These options are lower in fat and calories compared to red meat, providing essential nutrients without excessive saturated fats.
- Plant-Based Proteins: Incorporate plant-based proteins such as tofu, beans, or lentils into your meals. These sources offer protein without the saturated fat found in some animal products.

Mindful Cooking Techniques:

- Grilling and Baking: Opt for grilling or baking over frying to minimize added fats. These cooking methods retain flavors without the need for excessive oil, resulting in healthier and lighter dishes.

Portion Control:

- Practice portion control to manage calorie intake. Use smaller plates, be mindful of serving sizes, and listen to your body's hunger cues to avoid over consumption.

Balanced Ingredient Combinations:

- Fiber-Rich Foods: Integrate fiber-rich foods like whole grains, fruits, and vegetables into your meals. These additions provide bulk, promoting a feeling of fullness without contributing excess calories.
- Protein-Fiber Combo: Combine proteins with fiber to create satis-

fying and balanced meals. For instance, pair grilled chicken with a quinoa and vegetable salad for a meal that is both nutritious and filling.

Smart Snacking Choices:

- Nut and Seed Mixes: Create your own nut and seed mixes for snacking. These combinations provide healthy fats and proteins, curbing hunger without resorting to high-calorie snacks.
- Fresh Fruit Options: Choose fresh fruits for snacks instead of sugary alternatives. The natural sugars in fruits provide sweetness while offering essential vitamins and minerals, making for a wholesome and satisfying snack.

By incorporating these strategies, you not only reduce undesirable elements like fat, calories, sugar, and sodium but also enhance the nutritional quality of your meals. Balancing these factors promotes a healthier and more mindful approach to cooking and contributes to overall well-being.

Easy, Good Tasting, and Healthy Recipes for Two

Dive into a treasure trove of recipes designed for two, ensuring simplicity, taste, and nutrition. From breakfast to dessert, discover a variety of meals that cater to different tastes and preferences.

- Breakfast Recipes - Start your day right with a collection of quick, delicious, and nutritious breakfast recipes. From energizing smoothies to hearty breakfast bowls, find options that fit your morning routine.
- Lunch Recipes - Elevate your midday meals with easy-to-prepare lunch options. From vibrant salads to satisfying wraps, these recipes

strike the perfect balance between convenience and flavor.

- Dinner Recipes - Whip up savory and wholesome dinners in 30 minutes or less. Explore a diverse range of recipes that cater to various tastes, making weeknight dinners a breeze.
- Desserts - Satisfy your sweet tooth with delectable desserts that won't break the bank or your healthy eating goals. Indulge in guilt-free treats that are quick to prepare and delightful to the palate.
- Healthier Snack Ideas - Elevate your snack game with easy, healthy, and budget-friendly options. Discover snacks that are perfect for satisfying cravings between meals without compromising your nutritional goals.

Breakfast Recipes

Berry Blast Smoothie

Ingredients:

- 1 cup mixed berries (strawberries, blueberries, raspberries)
- 1 ripe banana
- 1/2 cup Greek yogurt
- 1/2 cup almond milk
- Ice cubes (optional)

Instructions:

- Combine mixed berries, banana, Greek yogurt, and almond milk in a blender.
- Blend until smooth and creamy.
- Add ice cubes if desired and blend again.
- Pour into a glass and enjoy your refreshing Berry Blast Smoothie!

Nutrition Facts (approximate)

- Calories: 250
- Protein: 12g
- Fat: 7g
- Carbohydrates: 40g
- Fiber: 7g
- Sugar: 23g

Overnight Oats with Nut Butter

Ingredients:

- 1/2 cup rolled oats
- 1/2 cup almond milk
- 1 tablespoon chia seeds
- 1 tablespoon nut butter (almond or peanut)
- 1 banana, sliced
- 1 tablespoon honey

Instructions:

- In a jar, combine rolled oats, almond milk, chia seeds, and nut butter. Stir well.
- Refrigerate overnight or for at least 4 hours.
- Before serving, top with sliced banana and a drizzle of honey.

Nutrition Facts (approximate)

- Calories: 380
- Protein: 11g

- Fat: 17g
- Carbohydrates: 48g
- Fiber: 10g
- Sugar: 14g

Veggie Omelet

Ingredients:

- 3 eggs
- 1/2 bell pepper, diced
- 1/2 cup spinach, chopped
- 1/4 cup cherry tomatoes, halved
- Salt and pepper to taste
- 1 tablespoon olive oil

Instructions:

- In a bowl, whisk the eggs until well beaten. Season with salt and pepper.
- Heat olive oil in a non-stick skillet over medium heat.
- Add bell pepper and cook until softened, then add spinach and cherry tomatoes.
- Pour the beaten eggs over the vegetables, swirling the pan to spread evenly.
- Allow the eggs to set around the edges, then gently lift the edges with a spatula to let the uncooked eggs flow underneath.
- When the omelet is mostly set but still slightly runny on top, fold it in half.
- Cook for an additional minute until the eggs are fully cooked.
- Slide the omelet onto a plate and serve.

Nutrition Facts (approximate)

- Calories: 300
- Protein: 18g
- Fat: 21g
- Carbohydrates: 10g
- Fiber: 3g
- Sugar: 6g

Avocado Toast with Poached Eggs

Ingredients:

- 2 slices whole-grain bread, toasted
- 1 ripe avocado, mashed
- 2 poached eggs
- Salt and pepper to taste
- Optional toppings: red pepper flakes, cherry tomatoes, or micro-greens

Instructions:

- Toast the whole-grain bread slices to your liking.
- Mash the ripe avocado and spread it evenly on the toasted bread.
- Top each slice with a poached egg.
- Season with salt and pepper, and add any optional toppings you prefer.
- Serve immediately for a delicious and nutritious breakfast.

Nutrition Facts (approximate)

- Calories: 400
- Protein: 15g
- Fat: 28g
- Carbohydrates: 28g
- Fiber: 12g
- Sugar: 3g

Greek Yogurt Parfait

Ingredients:

- 1 cup Greek yogurt
- 1/2 cup granola
- 1/2 cup mixed berries (strawberries, blueberries, raspberries)
- 1 tablespoon honey

Instructions:

- In a glass or bowl, layer Greek yogurt, granola, and mixed berries.
- Repeat the layers until the container is filled.
- Drizzle honey on top.
- Repeat the layering process for another parfait.
- Enjoy this simple and satisfying Greek Yogurt Parfait.

Nutrition Facts (approximate)

- Calories: 350
- Protein: 20g
- Fat: 12g
- Carbohydrates: 45g
- Fiber: 7g

- Sugar: 22g

Quinoa Breakfast Bowl

Ingredients:

- 1/2 cup cooked quinoa
- 1/2 cup almond milk
- 1 tablespoon chia seeds
- Sliced banana
- Handful of chopped nuts (e.g., almonds or walnuts)
- Drizzle of maple syrup (optional)

Instructions:

- In a bowl, combine cooked quinoa, almond milk, and chia seeds.
- Stir well and let it sit for a few minutes to allow the chia seeds to absorb the liquid.
- Top the quinoa mixture with sliced banana and chopped nuts.
- If desired, drizzle with maple syrup for sweetness.
- Mix everything together and enjoy this nutritious Quinoa Breakfast Bowl.

Nutrition Facts (approximate)

- Calories: 420
- Protein: 15g
- Fat: 18g
- Carbohydrates: 52g
- Fiber: 9g
- Sugar: 10g

Whole Grain Pancakes with Berries

Ingredients:

- 1 cup whole wheat flour
- 1 tablespoon baking powder
- 1 tablespoon honey
- 1 cup almond milk
- 1 egg
- 1 cup mixed berries (strawberries, blueberries, raspberries)
- Maple syrup for drizzling

Instructions:

- In a bowl, whisk together whole wheat flour, baking powder, honey, almond milk, and egg until well combined.
- Heat a non-stick skillet or griddle over medium heat.
- Pour 1/4 cup of batter onto the skillet for each pancake.
- Cook until bubbles form on the surface, then flip and cook until the other side is golden brown.
- Repeat until all the batter is used.
- Top the pancakes with mixed berries and drizzle with maple syrup.

Nutrition Facts (approximate)

- Calories: 320
- Protein: 10g
- Fat: 8g
- Carbohydrates: 55g
- Fiber: 10g
- Sugar: 12g

Peanut Butter Banana Toast

Ingredients:

- 2 slices whole-grain bread, toasted
- 2 tablespoons peanut butter
- 1 banana, sliced
- Drizzle of honey (optional)
- Sprinkle of chia seeds (optional)

Instructions:

- Toast the whole-grain bread slices.
- Spread peanut butter evenly on each slice.
- Arrange banana slices on top.
- If desired, drizzle honey over the bananas and sprinkle with chia seeds.
- Enjoy this quick and delicious Peanut Butter Banana Toast.

Nutrition Facts (approximate)

- Calories: 350
- Protein: 10g
- Fat: 18g
- Carbohydrates: 40g
- Fiber: 7g
- Sugar: 15g

Spinach and Feta Scramble

Ingredients:

- 3 eggs
- Handful of fresh spinach, chopped
- 2 tablespoons feta cheese, crumbled
- Salt and pepper to taste
- 1 teaspoon olive oil

Instructions:

- In a bowl, beat the eggs and season with salt and pepper.
- Heat olive oil in a skillet over medium heat.
- Add chopped spinach and cook until wilted.
- Pour the beaten eggs over the spinach.
- As the eggs start to set, gently stir, incorporating the spinach.
- Once the eggs are mostly cooked, add crumbled feta and continue stirring until fully cooked.
- Serve this nutritious Spinach and Feta Scramble warm.

Nutrition Facts (approximate)

- Calories: 280
- Protein: 17g
- Fat: 20g
- Carbohydrates: 7g
- Fiber: 2g
- Sugar: 2g

Blueberry Almond Overnight Oats
Ingredients:

- 1/2 cup rolled oats

- 1/2 cup almond milk
- 1/2 cup fresh blueberries
- 1 tablespoon almond butter
- 1 teaspoon chia seeds
- Drizzle of maple syrup (optional)

Instructions:

- In a jar, combine rolled oats, almond milk, blueberries, almond butter, and chia seeds.
- Stir well, ensuring all ingredients are evenly distributed.
- Refrigerate overnight or for at least 4 hours.
- Before serving, give the oats a good stir.
- If desired, drizzle with maple syrup for added sweetness.
- Enjoy your tasty and convenient Blueberry Almond Overnight Oats.

Nutrition Facts (approximate)

- Calories: 330
- Protein: 8g
- Fat: 15g
- Carbohydrates: 41g
- Fiber: 8g
- Sugar: 9g

Lunch Recipes

Chickpea and Vegetable Salad
Ingredients:

- 1 can chickpeas, drained and rinsed
- 1 cup cherry tomatoes, halved
- 1 cucumber, diced
- 1/2 cup feta cheese, crumbled
- 2 tablespoons olive oil
- 1 tablespoon lemon juice
- Salt and pepper to taste

Instructions:

- In a large bowl, combine chickpeas, cherry tomatoes, cucumber, and feta cheese.
- In a small bowl, whisk together olive oil, lemon juice, salt, and pepper.
- Drizzle the dressing over the salad and toss gently to combine.
- Serve immediately or refrigerate for later.

Nutrition Facts (approximate)

- Calories: 280
- Protein: 9g
- Fat: 15g
- Carbohydrates: 30g
- Fiber: 9g
- Sugar: 6g

Grilled Chicken Wrap

Ingredients:

- 2 boneless, skinless chicken breasts

- 4 whole-grain wraps
- 1 cup mixed greens
- 1 tomato, sliced
- 1/2 cucumber, sliced
- Greek yogurt dressing

Instructions:

- Season chicken breasts with salt and pepper. Grill until fully cooked.
- Slice grilled chicken into strips.
- Assemble wraps with chicken, mixed greens, tomato, cucumber, and a drizzle of Greek yogurt dressing.
- Roll up the wraps and serve.

Nutrition Facts (approximate)

- Calories: 400
- Protein: 30g
- Fat: 12g
- Carbohydrates: 45g
- Fiber: 8g
- Sugar: 5g

Quinoa Salad with Chickpeas and Mediterranean Veggies

Ingredients:

- 1 cup cooked quinoa
- 1 can chickpeas, drained and rinsed
- 1 cup cherry tomatoes, halved
- 1 cucumber, diced

- 1/4 cup red onion, finely chopped
- Kalamata olives, sliced
- Feta cheese, crumbled
- Olive oil and lemon juice dressing
- Fresh parsley, chopped

Instructions:

- In a large bowl, combine cooked quinoa, chickpeas, cherry tomatoes, cucumber, red onion, olives, and feta cheese.
- Drizzle with olive oil and lemon juice dressing.
- Toss the salad until well mixed.
- Garnish with fresh parsley before serving.

Nutrition Facts (approximate)

- Calories: 350
- Protein: 13g
- Fat: 15g
- Carbohydrates: 45g
- Fiber: 9g
- Sugar: 6g

Veggie Wrap with Hummus

Ingredients:

- Whole-grain wraps
- Hummus
- Baby spinach leaves
- Shredded carrots

- Sliced bell peppers (assorted colors)
- Cucumber, julienned
- Avocado, sliced

Instructions:

- Spread a generous layer of hummus on each whole-grain wrap.
- Layer baby spinach, shredded carrots, sliced bell peppers, cucumber, and avocado.
- Roll up the wraps and slice them in half.
- Secure with toothpicks if needed and enjoy a flavorful Veggie Wrap.

Nutrition Facts (approximate)

- Calories: 350
- Protein: 10g
- Fat: 12g
- Carbohydrates: 50g
- Fiber: 9g
- Sugar: 5g

Lentil and Vegetable Stir-Fry

Ingredients:

- 1 cup cooked lentils
- Broccoli florets
- Snap peas
- Carrots, julienned
- Bell peppers, sliced
- Garlic, minced

- Soy sauce
- Sesame oil
- Red pepper flakes (optional)

Instructions:

- In a wok or skillet, heat sesame oil over medium-high heat.
- Add minced garlic and stir-fry until fragrant.
- Add broccoli, snap peas, carrots, and bell peppers. Stir-fry until vegetables are tender-crisp.
- Add cooked lentils to the vegetables.
- Drizzle with soy sauce and toss to coat.
- Optional: Add red pepper flakes for some heat.
- Serve the Lentil and Vegetable Stir-Fry over brown rice or quinoa.

Nutrition Facts (approximate)

- Calories: 350
- Protein: 18g
- Fat: 8g
- Carbohydrates: 50g
- Fiber: 15g
- Sugar: 8g

Turkey and Avocado Wrap

Ingredients:

- Whole-grain wraps
- Turkey slices
- Avocado, sliced

- Tomato, sliced
- Lettuce leaves
- Greek yogurt dressing

Instructions:

- Lay out a whole-grain wrap and place turkey slices on it.
- Top with avocado slices, tomato slices, and lettuce leaves.
- Drizzle with Greek yogurt dressing.
- Roll up the wrap and slice it in half.
- Enjoy this delicious and protein-packed Turkey and Avocado Wrap.

Nutrition Facts (approximate)

- Calories: 380
- Protein: 25g
- Fat: 15g
- Carbohydrates: 35g
- Fiber: 7g
- Sugar: 5g

Caprese Salad with Balsamic Glaze

Ingredients:

- Fresh mozzarella balls
- Cherry tomatoes, halved
- Fresh basil leaves
- Balsamic glaze
- Olive oil
- Salt and pepper to taste

Instructions:

- Arrange fresh mozzarella balls and cherry tomato halves on a serving platter.
- Tuck fresh basil leaves between the mozzarella and tomatoes.
- Drizzle with balsamic glaze and olive oil.
- Season with salt and pepper to taste.
- Serve this classic Caprese Salad as a refreshing and light lunch.

Nutrition Facts (approximate)

- Calories: 250
- Protein: 12g
- Fat: 18g
- Carbohydrates: 10g
- Fiber: 2g
- Sugar: 6g

Chickpea and Avocado Salad
Ingredients:

- 1 can chickpeas, drained and rinsed
- Avocado, diced
- Red onion, finely chopped
- Cilantro, chopped
- Lime juice
- Salt and pepper to taste

Instructions:

- In a bowl, combine chickpeas, diced avocado, red onion, and cilantro.
- Squeeze fresh lime juice over the mixture.
- Season with salt and pepper to taste.
- Gently toss the ingredients until well combined.
- Serve this quick and tasty Chickpea and Avocado Salad.

Nutrition Facts (approximate)

- Calories: 320
- Protein: 9g
- Fat: 16g
- Carbohydrates: 38g
- Fiber: 14g
- Sugar: 6g

Grilled Chicken Caesar Salad

Ingredients:

- Grilled chicken breast, sliced
- Romaine lettuce, chopped
- Cherry tomatoes, halved
- Croutons
- Parmesan cheese, grated
- Caesar dressing

Instructions:

- In a large bowl, combine chopped romaine lettuce, grilled chicken slices, cherry tomatoes, croutons, and grated Parmesan cheese.
- Drizzle with Caesar dressing.

- Toss the salad until evenly coated.
- Serve this Grilled Chicken Caesar Salad for a satisfying and protein-rich lunch.

Nutrition Facts (approximate)

- Calories: 380
- Protein: 30g
- Fat: 18g
- Carbohydrates: 25g
- Fiber: 5g
- Sugar: 5g

Quinoa and Black Bean Bowl

Ingredients:

- 1 cup cooked quinoa
- 1 can black beans, drained and rinsed
- Corn kernels (fresh or frozen)
- Avocado, diced
- Salsa
- Fresh cilantro, chopped
- Lime wedges

Instructions:

- In a bowl, layer cooked quinoa, black beans, corn, and diced avocado.
- Top with salsa and fresh cilantro.
- Squeeze lime wedges over the bowl for extra flavor.
- Enjoy this Quinoa and Black Bean Bowl as a nutritious and satisfying

lunch.

Nutrition Facts (approximate)

- Calories: 400
- Protein: 18g
- Fat: 15g
- Carbohydrates: 55g
- Fiber: 15g
- Sugar: 3g

Dinner Recipes

Sheet Pan Salmon with Roasted Vegetables

Ingredients:

- 2 salmon fillets
- 1 cup broccoli florets
- 1 cup cherry tomatoes
- 1 bell pepper, sliced
- 2 tablespoons olive oil
- 1 teaspoon garlic powder
- 1 teaspoon dried oregano
- Salt and pepper to taste

Instructions:

- Preheat the oven to 400°F (200°C).
- Place salmon fillets in the center of a baking sheet.
- Surround the salmon with broccoli, cherry tomatoes, and sliced bell

pepper.

- Drizzle olive oil over the salmon and vegetables. Sprinkle garlic powder, dried oregano, salt, and pepper.
- Toss the vegetables to coat them in the oil and seasoning.
- Bake for 15-20 minutes or until the salmon is cooked through and flakes easily with a fork.
- Serve the salmon on a plate with roasted vegetables.

Nutrition Facts (approximate)

- Calories: 400
- Protein: 30g
- Fat: 25g
- Carbohydrates: 15g
- Fiber: 5g
- Sugar: 5g

Quinoa-Stuffed Bell Peppers

Ingredients:

- 2 bell peppers, halved and seeds removed
- 1 cup cooked quinoa
- 1 can black beans, drained and rinsed
- 1 cup corn kernels (fresh or frozen)
- 1 teaspoon cumin
- 1/2 teaspoon chili powder
- 1/2 cup shredded cheese (cheddar or Mexican blend)

Instructions:

- Preheat the oven to 375°F (190°C).
- In a bowl, mix cooked quinoa, black beans, corn, cumin, and chili powder.
- Stuff each bell pepper half with the quinoa mixture.
- Top with shredded cheese.
- Bake for 20-25 minutes or until peppers are tender.

Nutrition Facts (approximate)

- Calories: 300
- Protein: 15g
- Fat: 10g
- Carbohydrates: 40g
- Fiber: 8g
- Sugar: 5g

Lemon Garlic Shrimp Pasta

Ingredients:

- 8 oz whole wheat spaghetti
- 1 lb shrimp, peeled and deveined
- 3 cloves garlic, minced
- 1 lemon, zest and juice
- 2 tablespoons olive oil
- Cherry tomatoes, halved
- Spinach leaves
- Parmesan cheese, grated
- Salt and pepper to taste

Instructions:

- Cook whole wheat spaghetti according to package instructions.
- In a skillet, heat olive oil and sauté minced garlic until fragrant.
- Add shrimp and cook until pink.
- Stir in lemon zest, lemon juice, cherry tomatoes, and spinach.
- Toss with cooked spaghetti.
- Season with salt and pepper.
- Serve with grated Parmesan cheese.

Nutrition Facts (approximate)

- Calories: 450
- Protein: 30g
- Fat: 20g
- Carbohydrates: 40g
- Fiber: 6g
- Sugar: 5g

Baked Chicken and Vegetables

Ingredients:

- 4 boneless, skinless chicken breasts
- Baby potatoes, halved
- Carrots, peeled and sliced
- Broccoli florets
- Olive oil
- Garlic powder, paprika, salt, and pepper to taste

Instructions:

- Preheat the oven to 400°F (200°C).

- Place chicken breasts on a baking sheet.
- Surround with halved baby potatoes, sliced carrots, and broccoli.
- Drizzle with olive oil and sprinkle with garlic powder, paprika, salt, and pepper.
- Bake for 25-30 minutes or until chicken is cooked through and vegetables are tender.

Nutrition Facts (approximate)

- Calories: 380
- Protein: 35g
- Fat: 15g
- Carbohydrates: 30g
- Fiber: 7g
- Sugar: 3g

Vegetarian Stir-Fried Tofu and Vegetables

Ingredients:

- 14 oz firm tofu, pressed and cubed
- Broccoli florets
- Bell peppers, sliced
- Snow peas
- Carrots, julienned
- Soy sauce, ginger, and garlic for stir-frying
- Brown rice or quinoa for serving

Instructions:

- In a wok or skillet, stir-fry cubed tofu until golden.

- Add broccoli, bell peppers, snow peas, and carrots.
- Stir in soy sauce, ginger, and garlic.
- Continue stir-frying until vegetables are tender.
- Serve over brown rice or quino

Nutrition Facts (approximate)

- Calories: 350
- Protein: 20g
- Fat: 18g
- Carbohydrates: 30g
- Fiber: 10g
- Sugar: 5g

Turkey and Vegetable Stuffed Peppers

Ingredients:

- Bell peppers, halved and seeds removed
- 1 lb ground turkey
- Quinoa, cooked
- Black beans, drained and rinsed
- Corn kernels (fresh or frozen)
- Tomato sauce
- Chili powder, cumin, salt, and pepper to taste
- Shredded cheese for topping

Instructions:

- Preheat the oven to 375°F (190°C).
- Brown ground turkey in a skillet.

- In a bowl, mix cooked quinoa, black beans, corn, and tomato sauce.
- Season with chili powder, cumin, salt, and pepper.
- Stuff bell peppers with the turkey and quinoa mixture.
- Top with shredded cheese.
- Bake for 25-30 minutes or until peppers are tender.

Nutrition Facts (approximate)

- Calories: 320
- Protein: 25g
- Fat: 12g
- Carbohydrates: 30g
- Fiber: 7g
- Sugar: 6g

Teriyaki Salmon with Stir-Fried Vegetables

Ingredients:

- 4 salmon fillets
- Teriyaki sauce
- Broccoli florets
- Snap peas
- Carrots, sliced
- Brown rice for serving

Instructions:

- Marinate salmon fillets in teriyaki sauce.
- In a pan, sear salmon until cooked through.
- In the same pan, stir-fry broccoli, snap peas, and carrots.

- Serve the teriyaki salmon over brown rice with stir-fried vegetables.

Nutrition Facts (approximate)

- Calories: 420
- Protein: 30g
- Fat: 20g
- Carbohydrates: 25g
- Fiber: 6g
- Sugar: 10g

Lentil and Vegetable Curry

Ingredients:

- 1 cup dried lentils, cooked
- Mixed vegetables (e.g., cauliflower, peas, carrots)
- Onion, chopped
- Garlic, minced
- Curry powder, cumin, coriander, turmeric
- Coconut milk
- Tomato sauce
- Brown rice for serving

Instructions:

- Sauté onion and garlic in a pot until softened.
- Add mixed vegetables and cook until slightly tender.
- Stir in cooked lentils, curry powder, cumin, coriander, and turmeric.
- Pour in coconut milk and tomato sauce.
- Simmer until vegetables are cooked.

- Serve the lentil and vegetable curry over brown rice.

Nutrition Facts (approximate)

- Calories: 350
- Protein: 18g
- Fat: 15g
- Carbohydrates: 40g
- Fiber: 12g
- Sugar: 6g

Grilled Vegetable and Quinoa Bowl

Ingredients:

- Zucchini, sliced
- Eggplant, sliced
- Red onion, sliced
- Bell peppers, sliced
- Quinoa, cooked
- Balsamic vinaigrette dressing
- Fresh basil, chopped

Instructions:

- Grill zucchini, eggplant, red onion, and bell peppers until charred.
- In a bowl, combine grilled vegetables with cooked quinoa.
- Drizzle with balsamic vinaigrette dressing.
- Garnish with fresh basil.

Nutrition Facts (approximate)

- Calories: 320
- Protein: 12g
- Fat: 15g
- Carbohydrates: 40g
- Fiber: 8g
- Sugar: 5g

Chicken and Broccoli Stir-Fry

Ingredients:

- 1 lb chicken breast, sliced
- Broccoli florets
- Soy sauce, ginger, and garlic for stir-frying
- Brown rice for serving

Instructions:

- Stir-fry sliced chicken in a wok until cooked through.
- Add broccoli florets and continue stir-frying.
- Season with soy sauce, ginger, and garlic.
- Serve the chicken and broccoli stir-fry over brown rice.

Nutrition Facts (approximate)

- Calories: 340
- Protein: 30g
- Fat: 10g
- Carbohydrates: 30g
- Fiber: 7g
- Sugar: 4g

Mediterranean Chickpea Salad

Ingredients:

- 2 cans chickpeas, drained and rinsed
- Cucumber, diced
- Cherry tomatoes, halved
- Red onion, finely chopped
- Kalamata olives, sliced
- Feta cheese, crumbled
- Olive oil and lemon juice dressing
- Fresh oregano, chopped

Instructions:

- In a bowl, combine chickpeas, cucumber, cherry tomatoes, red onion, olives, and feta cheese.
- Drizzle with olive oil and lemon juice dressing.
- Toss the salad until well mixed.
- Garnish with fresh oregano before serving.

Nutrition Facts (approximate)

- Calories: 280
- Protein: 10g
- Fat: 15g
- Carbohydrates: 30g
- Fiber: 8g
- Sugar: 6g

Spaghetti Aglio e Olio with Shrimp

Ingredients:

- 8 oz whole wheat spaghetti
- 1/2 cup olive oil
- 4 cloves garlic, thinly sliced
- Red pepper flakes (optional)
- Shrimp, peeled and deveined
- Fresh parsley, chopped
- Parmesan cheese, grated

Instructions:

- Cook whole wheat spaghetti according to package instructions.
- In a pan, heat olive oil and sauté thinly sliced garlic until golden.
- Add red pepper flakes if desired.
- Add shrimp and cook until pink.
- Toss cooked spaghetti in the garlic and oil mixture.
- Garnish with fresh parsley and grated Parmesan cheese.

Nutrition Facts (approximate)

- Calories: 400
- Protein: 25g
- Fat: 20g
- Carbohydrates: 35g
- Fiber: 5g
- Sugar: 3g

Desserts

Mixed Berry Yogurt Popsicles

Ingredients:

- 1 cup mixed berries (strawberries, blueberries, raspberries)
- 2 cups Greek yogurt
- 2 tablespoons honey

Instructions:

- In a blender, puree the mixed berries until smooth.
- In a bowl, mix Greek yogurt and honey.
- Layer the berry puree and yogurt mixture in popsicle molds.
- Use a stick to swirl the layers for a marbled effect.
- Insert popsicle sticks and freeze for at least 4 hours or until firm.
- Run molds under warm water to release popsicles and enjoy your Mixed Berry Yogurt Popsicle!

Nutrition Facts (approximate)

- Calories: 90
- Protein: 6g
- Fat: 2g
- Carbohydrates: 15g
- Fiber: 2g
- Sugar: 11g

Dark Chocolate-Dipped Strawberries

Ingredients:

- Fresh strawberries

- Dark chocolate (70% cocoa or higher)

Instructions:

- Melt dark chocolate in a microwave-safe bowl in 30-second intervals, stirring between each interval.
- Dip each strawberry into the melted chocolate, covering half or two-thirds of the berry.
- Place dipped strawberries on a parchment-lined tray.
- Allow the chocolate to set, either at room temperature or in the refrigerator.

Nutrition Facts (approximate)

- Calories: 50 (per strawberry)
- Protein: 1g
- Fat: 3g
- Carbohydrates: 6g
- Fiber: 2g
- Sugar: 3g

Fruit Salad with Honey-Lime Dressing

Ingredients:

- Assorted fresh fruits (strawberries, pineapple, kiwi, grapes)
- Honey
- Lime juice
- Fresh mint leaves

Instructions:

- Chop fresh fruits into bite-sized pieces and place in a bowl.
- In a small bowl, whisk together honey and lime juice.
- Drizzle the honey-lime dressing over the fruit.
- Toss gently to coat.
- Garnish with fresh mint leaves.

Nutrition Facts (approximate)

- Calories: 80
- Protein: 1g
- Fat: 0g
- Carbohydrates: 20g
- Fiber: 3g
- Sugar: 15g

Chocolate Avocado Mousse

Ingredients:

- 2 ripe avocados
- 1/4 cup cocoa powder
- 1/4 cup maple syrup
- 1 teaspoon vanilla extract
- Pinch of salt
- Fresh berries for topping

Instructions:

- In a blender, combine avocados, cocoa powder, maple syrup, vanilla extract, and a pinch of salt.
- Blend until smooth and creamy.

- Refrigerate for at least 30 minutes.
- Serve chilled, topped with fresh berries.

Nutrition Facts (approximate)

- Calories: 180
- Protein: 2g
- Fat: 14g
- Carbohydrates: 18g
- Fiber: 6g
- Sugar: 8g

Greek Yogurt Parfait with Granola and Berries

Ingredients:

- Greek yogurt
- Granola
- Mixed berries (strawberries, blueberries, raspberries)
- Honey

Instructions:

- In a glass, layer Greek yogurt, granola, and mixed berries.
- Repeat the layers until the glass is filled.
- Drizzle with honey.
- Serve this simple and healthy Greek Yogurt Parfait.

Nutrition Facts (approximate)

- Calories: 250

- Protein: 15g
- Fat: 8g
- Carbohydrates: 35g
- Fiber: 4g
- Sugar: 15g

Baked Apples with Cinnamon and Walnuts

Ingredients:

- Apples, cored and halved
- Cinnamon
- Chopped walnuts
- Maple syrup
- Greek yogurt for serving

Instructions:

- Preheat the oven to 375°F (190°C).
- Place cored and halved apples on a baking sheet.
- Sprinkle with cinnamon and chopped walnuts.
- Drizzle with maple syrup.
- Bake for 20-25 minutes or until apples are tender.
- Serve with a dollop of Greek yogurt.

Nutrition Facts (approximate)

- Calories: 180
- Protein: 2g
- Fat: 8g
- Carbohydrates: 30g

- Fiber: 6g
- Sugar: 20g

Mango Coconut Chia Pudding

Ingredients:

- 1/4 cup chia seeds
- 1 cup coconut milk
- 1 ripe mango, diced
- Toasted coconut flakes for garnish

Instructions:

- In a jar, mix chia seeds and coconut milk.
- Refrigerate for at least 2 hours or overnight.
- Layer diced mango over the chia pudding.
- Garnish with toasted coconut flakes.

Nutrition Facts (approximate)

- Calories: 220
- Protein: 4g
- Fat: 12g
- Carbohydrates: 26g
- Fiber: 8g
- Sugar: 14g

Banana Ice Cream

Ingredients:

- Ripe bananas, sliced and frozen
- Optional toppings: nuts, dark chocolate chips, shredded coconut

Instructions:

- Blend frozen banana slices in a food processor until creamy.
- Optional: Add toppings like nuts, dark chocolate chips, or shredded coconut.
- Serve immediately for a healthy and creamy Banana Ice Cream.

Nutrition Facts (approximate)

- Calories: 120 (per cup)
- Protein: 2g
- Fat: 1g
- Carbohydrates: 30g
- Fiber: 4g
- Sugar: 16g

Berry and Almond Crisp

Ingredients:

- Mixed berries (strawberries, blueberries, raspberries)
- Almond flour
- Rolled oats
- Maple syrup
- Sliced almonds

Instructions:

- In a bowl, mix mixed berries with a bit of almond flour.
- In a separate bowl, combine rolled oats, almond flour, and maple syrup.
- Spread the berry mixture in a baking dish and top with the oat mixture.
- Sprinkle sliced almonds on top.
- Bake at 350°F (175°C) for 25-30 minutes or until golden.

Nutrition Facts (approximate)

- Calories: 220
- Protein: 5g
- Fat: 8g
- Carbohydrates: 35g
- Fiber: 6g
- Sugar: 16g

Dark Chocolate Dipped Strawberries with Toppings

Ingredients:

- Fresh strawberries
- Dark chocolate, melted
- Chopped nuts or shredded coconut for coating

Instructions:

- Dip each strawberry into melted dark chocolate.
- Optional: Roll the chocolate-covered strawberries in chopped nuts or shredded coconut.
- Place on parchment paper and let the chocolate set.

- Enjoy these indulgent Dark Chocolate Dipped Strawberries.

Nutrition Facts (approximate)

- Calories: 60 (per strawberry, without additional toppings)
- Protein: 1g
- Fat: 4g
- Carbohydrates: 7g
- Fiber: 2g
- Sugar: 4g

Healthier Snack Ideas

Trail Mix with Nuts and Dried Fruit

Ingredients:

- 1/2 cup almonds
- 1/2 cup walnuts
- 1/4 cup pumpkin seeds
- 1/4 cup dried cranberries
- 1/4 cup dried apricots, chopped

Instructions:

- In a bowl, combine almonds, walnuts, pumpkin seeds, dried cranberries, and chopped dried apricots.
- Toss the ingredients until well mixed.
- Portion into snack-sized containers for easy grab-and-go access.
- Enjoy your homemade Trail Mix for a nutritious snack!

Nutrition Facts (approximate)

- Calories: 200
- Protein: 5g
- Fat: 15g
- Carbohydrates: 15g
- Fiber: 3g
- Sugar: 8g

Hummus & Veggie Sticks

Ingredients:

- Hummus (store-bought or homemade)
- Carrot sticks
- Cucumber slices
- Bell pepper strips

Instructions:

- Cut vegetables into sticks or slices.
- Serve with hummus for a tasty and satisfying snack.

Nutrition Facts (approximate)

- Calories: 150
- Protein: 5g
- Fat: 9g
- Carbohydrates: 15g
- Fiber: 6g
- Sugar: 3g

Greek Yogurt and Berry Parfait

Ingredients:

- Greek yogurt
- Mixed berries (blueberries, strawberries, raspberries)
- Granola
- Honey

Instructions:

- In a bowl or glass, layer Greek yogurt, mixed berries, and granola.
- Drizzle with honey for sweetness.
- Enjoy this protein-packed and flavorful Greek Yogurt and Berry Parfait.

Nutrition Facts (approximate)

- Calories: 250
- Protein: 20g
- Fat: 10g
- Carbohydrates: 25g
- Fiber: 5g
- Sugar: 15g

Veggie Sticks with Hummus

Ingredients:

- Carrot sticks
- Cucumber slices
- Bell pepper strips

- Hummus for dipping

Instructions:

- Slice carrots, cucumber, and bell pepper into sticks or strips.
- Serve with a side of hummus for a crunchy and satisfying snack.

Nutrition Facts (approximate)

- Calories: 100
- Protein: 3g
- Fat: 7g
- Carbohydrates: 10g
- Fiber: 4g
- Sugar: 3g

Almond Butter and Banana Slices

Ingredients:

- Almond butter
- Banana, sliced

Instructions:

- Spread almond butter on banana slices.
- Enjoy this simple and energy-boosting Almond Butter and Banana snack.

Nutrition Facts (approximate)

- Calories: 180
- Protein: 4g
- Fat: 14g
- Carbohydrates: 12g
- Fiber: 3g
- Sugar: 6g

Trail Mix with Nuts and Dried Fruit

Ingredients:

- Mixed nuts (almonds, walnuts, cashews)
- Dried fruit (apricots, cranberries, raisins)
- Dark chocolate chips

Instructions:

- Mix nuts, dried fruit, and dark chocolate chips in a bowl.
- Portion into small snack-sized bags for a convenient on-the-go option.

Nutrition Facts (approximate)

- Calories: 200
- Protein: 5g
- Fat: 15g
- Carbohydrates: 15g
- Fiber: 3g
- Sugar: 8g

Rice Cake with Avocado and Cherry Tomatoes

Ingredients:

- Brown rice cake
- Avocado, mashed
- Cherry tomatoes, halved
- Sprinkle of sea salt

Instructions:

- Spread mashed avocado on a brown rice cake.
- Top with halved cherry tomatoes and a sprinkle of sea salt.
- Enjoy this light and satisfying Rice Cake with Avocado.

Nutrition Facts (approximate)

- Calories: 150
- Protein: 3g
- Fat: 9g
- Carbohydrates: 15g
- Fiber: 4g
- Sugar: 1g

Cottage Cheese with Pineapple Chunks

Ingredients:

- Cottage cheese
- Fresh pineapple chunks

Instructions:

- Combine cottage cheese with fresh pineapple chunks.
- This sweet and savory combination makes for a protein-rich snack.

Nutrition Facts (approximate)

- Calories: 150
- Protein: 14g
- Fat: 6g
- Carbohydrates: 12g
- Fiber: 1g
- Sugar: 8g

Edamame with Sea Salt

Ingredients:

- Edamame (steamed or boiled)
- Sea salt

Instructions:

- Steam or boil edamame until tender.
- Sprinkle with sea salt for a nutritious and addictive snack.

Nutrition Facts (approximate)

- Calories: 150
- Protein: 13g
- Fat: 8g
- Carbohydrates: 8g
- Fiber: 4g

- Sugar: 2g

Apple Slices with Almond Butter

Ingredients:

- Apple, sliced
- Almond butter

Instructions:

- Spread almond butter on apple slices.
- This combination of fiber and healthy fats makes for a satisfying snack.

Nutrition Facts (approximate)

- Calories: 200
- Protein: 3g
- Fat: 11g
- Carbohydrates: 26g
- Fiber: 6g
- Sugar: 17g

Quinoa and Black Bean Salad

Ingredients:

- Cooked quinoa
- Black beans, drained and rinsed
- Corn kernels

- Cherry tomatoes, halved
- Cilantro, chopped
- Lime juice
- Salt and pepper

Instructions:

- Mix cooked quinoa, black beans, corn, cherry tomatoes, and cilantro.
- Drizzle with lime juice and season with salt and pepper.
- Enjoy this protein-packed Quinoa and Black Bean Salad.

Nutrition Facts (approximate)

- Calories: 180
- Protein: 7g
- Fat: 3g
- Carbohydrates: 32g
- Fiber: 6g
- Sugar: 4g

Whole Grain Crackers with Tuna Salad

Ingredients:

- Whole grain crackers
- Canned tuna, drained
- Greek yogurt
- Diced cucumber and cherry tomatoes
- Dill and black pepper

Instructions:

- Mix canned tuna with Greek yogurt, diced cucumber, cherry tomatoes, dill, and black pepper.
- Serve on whole grain crackers for a satisfying and protein-rich snack.

Nutrition Facts (approximate)

- Calories: 250
- Protein: 15g
- Fat: 10g
- Carbohydrates: 25g
- Fiber: 5g
- Sugar: 3g

Frozen Grapes

Ingredients:

- Grapes, washed and frozen

Instructions:

- Wash grapes and freeze them.
- Enjoy these refreshing and naturally sweet Frozen Grapes as a cool snack.

Nutrition Facts (approximate)

- Calories: 100
- Protein: 1g
- Fat: 0g

- Carbohydrates: 25g
- Fiber: 2g
- Sugar: 20g

All of the recipes listed above provide a variety of easy, healthy, and budget-friendly recipes for breakfast, lunch, dinner, desserts, and snacks. Enjoy delicious meals designed for two without breaking the bank or compromising on nutritional goals. Enjoy!

Let's dive into Chapter 5, "Creating the Lifestyle Change: Routines and Schedules," with a practical and helpful approach.

5

Creating the Lifestyle Change: Routines and Schedules

This chapter empowers you to make the most of your time by developing effective daily routines and schedules, ultimately enhancing productivity, and providing you with more time for the things that really matter.

Identifying and Reducing Time Wasters

In this section, discover practical strategies to identify and eliminate time-wasting activities from your daily life. Learn to distinguish between tasks that contribute to your goals and those that hinder progress, enabling you to streamline your efforts and focus on what truly matters.

- SMART Goal Setting: Make your goals Specific, Measurable, Achievable, Relevant, and Time-bound. This approach provides clarity, enabling you to stay focused and measure your progress effectively.
- Mindful Social Media Engagement: Instead of mindlessly scrolling through social media, allocate specific time slots for these activities.

Engage with intentionality and consider unfollowing accounts that don't add value to your life.

- Time Blocking: Divide your day into time blocks dedicated to specific activities. Whether it's work, leisure, or personal development, assigning time blocks ensures a disciplined approach to your daily schedule.
- Delegation Excellence: Recognize that you don't have to do everything yourself. Delegate tasks that others can handle, empowering you to focus on responsibilities that align with your expertise and priorities.
- The Art of Saying No: Cultivate the ability to decline commitments that don't align with your current goals or may overwhelm your schedule. Saying no is a powerful tool for preserving your time and energy.
- Minimalist Workspaces: Declutter both your physical and digital workspaces. A minimalist environment minimizes distractions, enhances clarity of thought, and fosters a more productive atmosphere.
- Themed Work Sessions: Group similar tasks into themed work sessions. For instance, designate specific times for emails, meetings, and creative work. This approach minimizes mental shifts, boosting overall efficiency.
- Regular Time Audits: Conduct regular time audits to assess how you spend each hour. Identify patterns, recognize time-wasting habits, and adjust your routines accordingly to align with your overarching goals.
- Boundaries for Well-being: Establish boundaries to protect your well-being. Define specific times for work, family, and personal activities, ensuring that one aspect of your life doesn't encroach upon the other.

By implementing these strategies, you'll develop a keen awareness of time-wasting habits and gain the tools needed to redirect your focus toward activities that bring fulfillment and joy to your life.

Creating a Daily Schedule for Monday-Friday

Unlock the secrets to crafting a tailored and efficient schedule for your weekdays. This subsection provides a guide to structuring your day, incorporating dedicated time blocks for work, exercise, meals, and relaxation. By following these guidelines, you'll optimize your daily routine to achieve a balance that suits your lifestyle, productivity, and well-being:

- Strategic Goal Setting: Begin your week by setting clear, strategic goals. Understand your overarching objectives, both short-term and long-term. Break these down into actionable tasks that can be distributed across the week.
- Morning Rituals for Productivity: Establish a consistent morning routine that jumpstarts your day on a positive note. Incorporate activities that contribute to your well-being, such as exercise, meditation, or a nutritious breakfast. This sets a tone of productivity and focus.
- Prioritize Daily Tasks: Identify the most critical tasks for each day. Prioritize based on urgency and importance, ensuring that your schedule revolves around accomplishing key objectives.
- Time Blocking Mastery: Implement time blocking to allocate specific periods to different types of activities. For example, reserve the morning for deep work, midday for meetings, and late afternoon for administrative tasks. Stick to these designated blocks to enhance focus and efficiency.
- Strategic Breaks: Schedule short breaks strategically throughout the day. These breaks serve as essential pauses, allowing you to

recharge and maintain sustained focus during work periods.

- Lunch and Midday Reset: Designate a specific time for lunch and a midday reset. Step away from your workspace, enjoy a nourishing meal, and engage in activities that help clear your mind, setting the stage for increased afternoon productivity.

- Flexibility for the Unforeseen: Acknowledge that unforeseen events may arise. Allow flexibility in your schedule to accommodate unexpected tasks or challenges without derailing your entire plan.

- Evening Wind-Down Ritual: Establish an evening wind-down ritual to signal the end of your workday. Reflect on your achievements, plan for the next day, and engage in relaxing activities that transition your mind from work mode to rest.

- Realistic Time frames: Set realistic time frames for each task. Avoid over committing, as this can lead to stress and a compromised quality of work. Be honest about the time required for each activity.

- Digital Detox Before Bed: Introduce a digital detox period before bedtime. Minimize exposure to screens, allowing your mind to unwind and promoting better sleep quality.

- Consistency as a Habit: Strive for consistency in your daily schedule. Consistency forms habits, making it easier to adhere to your routine over time. Regularity contributes to a sense of predictability and stability.

- Reflect and Adapt: Regularly reflect on the effectiveness of your daily schedule. Identify areas for improvement and adapt your routine to align with evolving priorities, energy levels, and external circumstances.

By implementing these guidelines, you'll develop a daily schedule that not only enhances your productivity but also promotes a healthy work-life balance. Stick to your routine, stay adaptable, and enjoy the positive impact on your overall well-being.

Tips to Relieve Stress

Navigating the demands of a busy can be challenging, but incorporating stress-relief strategies into your daily routine is essential for overall well-being. Explore these practical and accessible tips to alleviate stress and cultivate a happier, healthier lifestyle:

- Mindful Breathing: Incorporate moments of mindful breathing into your day. Take short breaks to focus on your breath, inhaling deeply and exhaling slowly. This simple practice can provide immediate relaxation.
- Daily Gratitude Practice: Cultivate gratitude by reflecting on positive aspects of your life daily. Whether through journaling or mental acknowledgment, expressing gratitude helps shift focus to positive elements, reducing stress.
- Establish Boundaries: Set clear boundaries between work and personal life. Define specific periods for work-related activities and allocate dedicated time for family, self-care, and leisure. Creating boundaries promotes balance.
- Physical Activity Breaks: Integrate short bursts of physical activity throughout your day. Whether it's a quick walk, stretching exercises, or a brief workout, physical activity releases endorphins, promoting stress relief.
- Connect with Nature: Spend time in nature whenever possible. Take a stroll in a nearby park, enjoy a lunch outdoors, or simply appreciate the natural beauty around you. Nature has a calming effect on the mind.
- Mindful Eating: Practice mindful eating by savoring each bite and paying attention to your body's hunger and fullness cues. This approach not only supports healthy eating but also fosters a mindful, stress-free relationship with food.

- Technology Detox: Designate specific periods for a technology detox. Disconnect from screens, especially before bedtime, to reduce digital-related stress and improve sleep quality.
- Creative Outlets: Engage in creative activities that bring joy, whether it's painting, writing, gardening, or playing a musical instrument. Creative outlets provide an emotional release and a sense of accomplishment.
- Social Connections: Foster meaningful social connections. Schedule regular time with friends or family, even if it's through virtual means. Social support is a powerful antidote to stress.
- Mind-Body Practices: Explore mind-body practices like yoga or meditation. These techniques promote relaxation, mindfulness, and a sense of inner calm.
- Quality Sleep Routine: Prioritize a consistent sleep routine. Create a calming pre-sleep ritual, avoid stimulants before bedtime, and ensure your sleep environment is conducive to restful sleep.
- Delegate Responsibilities: Recognize when you need assistance and delegate responsibilities. Whether at work or home, sharing tasks with others can lighten your load and reduce stress.
- Laugh and Have Fun: Incorporate laughter and fun into your daily life. Watch a funny movie, share jokes with friends, or engage in activities that bring genuine joy.
- Deep Tissue Massage or Relaxing Bath: Treat yourself to a deep tissue massage or a relaxing bath with essential oils. Physical relaxation can have a positive impact on mental well-being.
- Express Yourself: Find healthy ways to express your thoughts and emotions. Whether through journaling, talking to a friend, or seeking professional support, expressing yourself is a vital stress management tool.

Incorporating these practical tips into your daily routine can contribute to a significant reduction in stress levels. Experiment with different strategies to discover what works best for you and prioritize self-care as an integral part of your overall health and happiness.

6

Conclusion

In wrapping up our exploration of "Healthy Living for the Midlife Woman: Exercising and Eating Healthy on a Budget," let's focus on actionable takeaways. This guide is more than a read—it's a toolkit for change. We've covered staying active, budget-friendly healthy eating, and crafting a balanced routine. Now, it's about putting this knowledge into practice.

This isn't the end; it's a starting point for your ongoing journey to a healthier, happier you. Take these practical tips as your compass for navigating midlife challenges. Embrace small steps as progress and apply the strategies consistently. Your commitment to self-care is an investment in your future well-being.

Whether it's mindful breathing, gratitude rituals, or squeezing in physical activity, make these practices a daily habit. Establish clear boundaries between work and personal life, connect with nature, and unleash your creativity. Progress matters more than perfection, so celebrate every achievement.

If this guide resonates with you, leave a review on Amazon. Your insights could be the guidance someone needs.

This isn't a farewell but a new beginning. Here's to your health, happiness, and the promising chapters ahead. You have the power to thrive in every season of life—keep moving forward.